Food Allergy

FOOD ALLERGY

A Primer for People

SECOND EDITION

by
S. Allan Bock, M.D.

With a Historical Preface by
Charles D. May, M.D.

VANTAGE PRESS
New York / Atlanta
Los Angeles / Chicago

REVISED EDITION

Published by Vantage Press, Inc.
516 West 34th Street, New York, New York 10001

Manufactured in the United States of America
ISBN: 0-533-07562-9

Library of Congress Catalog Card No.: 87-90159

To my parents,
who supported and encouraged me
throughout my education

Contents

Preface to Second Edition

Since this primer was first written, there have been a number of important advances in this field. The author and his colleagues in other parts of the country have continued to find that the double-blind food challenge is the "gold standard" for proving that any individual is having a reaction to a particular food. New symptoms have begun to be examined. It is now more clear than ever that some children with eczema need to be evaluated for food allergy. Migraine headaches are receiving a critical appraisal with respect to their association with food ingestion. Adverse reactions to multiple foods and behavioral reactions to foods continue to be quite rare. It is more and more clear that many adverse reactions, including severe ones in young children, may be "outgrown" and that *careful* rechallenge at regular intervals is an important part of the treatment of patients with confirmed adverse reactions to food. Of course, some of the older food allergy fads have fallen by the wayside to be replaced by new, equally unproven ones.

I hope that the reader who has covered this ground before will be pleased with the new information and that the reader who is new to this territory will be helped to understand this field, which is often muddled by the extravagant claims found in most lay publications about food allergy.

Acknowledgments

Special thanks go to Charles D. May, M.D., with whom I have collaborated during the last twelve years and who generously contributed the historical preface of this volume. I would like to thank all of the people at the National Jewish Center for Immunology and Respiratory Medicine who helped us make the kinds of observations discussed here. And, finally, I would like to thank my friends and patients who urged me to undertake this project.

Historical Preface

Many articles on food allergy have appeared in newspapers and magazines in recent years that would lead the reader to believe almost any symptom known to man may be caused by an allergic reaction to some food. The articles usually go on to state that physicians disagree about the symptoms and management of food allergy. Readers are left with the impression that food allergy is too complicated and controversial to expect satisfactory diagnosis and treatment from most physicians—the reader feels confused.

In this primer, an allergist presents an uncomplicated approach to management of food allergy that practical experience has shown to result in accurate diagnosis and successful treatment in almost every case—confusion is dispelled.

The rationale of this helpful approach to food allergy will become apparent if the reasons controversy and confusion came to permeate the subject are recognized. The explanations come from three sources: 1) the history of the development of knowledge about food allergy; 2) the different ways opinions on the causes of illness are adopted; and 3) how the nature of illness is viewed in the broadest sense. Food allergy offers an exceptional illustration of the interplay of these factors in influencing the way we deal with disturbances in health.

HISTORICAL DEVELOPMENT

Allergy as a cause of disease was not recognized until as late as 1902, when two French scientists discovered the phenomenon under picturesque circumstances. The prince of Monaco at the time, Albert I, had an interest in oceanography, which he pursued with cruises on his yacht. He regularly took scientists with him to study marine life. On a voyage in the summer of 1901, Charles Richet and Paul Portier of the University of Paris undertook to isolate a poison from the tentacles of a gelatinous floating creature called the Portugese man-of-war, which seemed to kill its prey by means of this poison. They succeeded in making a toxic extract from the tentacles and then determined the dose required to kill some pigeons they had brought on board. In the course of their studies, completed in Paris in 1902, they found that if animals that had exhibited no symptoms from an injection of a small dose of the extract were given another equally small dose a week later, the animals developed severe, often fatal reactions. The animals had developed a changed reaction, a sensitivity, to the extract from the initial injection, a situation Richet and Portier called anaphylaxis and is now generally known as allergy. In 1913, Richet was awarded the Nobel Prize for his discovery and further studies.

Early in the course of his studies, Richet turned his attention to the question of whether allergy might be the explanation for severe reactions that had been observed in some people when they ate eggs and when some infants were fed cows' milk instead of their mothers' milk. His son, Charles Richet, Jr., worked in the same laboratories, becoming particularly involved with this question, and, along with his associates, demonstrated that specific allergic sensitivity to foods could be developed in experimental animals by feeding various foodstuffs. He found that allergic reactions occurred on subsequent reexposure.

The importance of these events for the subsequent course of food allergy is that Charles Richet, Jr., and Albert H. Rowe, a prominent allergist in San Francisco, California, collaborated in publication of a paper in a reputable French medical journal in 1930. They reported their clinical impressions that some persons they believed to have allergic reactions to foods exhibited many subjective complaints, such as headache and nervousness and behavioral disturbances. Rowe later elaborated upon his experience in a monograph.

The prestige of these authors and the appeal of food allergy as an explanation for many complaints bothersome to both physicians and patients led to widespread adoption of their opinion, and enthusiastic disciples of these men are prevalent. Unfortunately, the nervous and other symptoms ascribed to food allergy through Richet and Rowe's clinical impressions are the same complaints of psychologic nature heard from neurotic persons.

Currently, we are aware that clinical impressions may be the most untrustworthy because the best of physicians may be deceived by his or her preconceived ideas, bias, or prejudice. We have learned that steps must be taken to make observations objectively if error in clinical observations is to be avoided. This is particularly true where vague and subjective symptoms are concerned, as with the claims about food allergy being a cause of symptoms of this sort. The separation of psychological symptoms from manifestations of an allergic reaction to a food can be accomplished by a blind food challenge. In this procedure, neither patient nor physician knows what food is being tested because the food is hidden in another food or in opaque capsules. The details will be described fully in chapter 5.

When this procedure was followed in recent studies, the multitudinous bizarre, vague, and subjective symptoms often ascribed to food allergy by patients and physicians were not seen in response to eating the suspected foods, indicating the complaints were psychologic in origin. Instead, when a reaction was produced, the symptoms were those known to be characteristic of genuine allergic disorders.

WAYS OF ADOPTING OPINIONS

Certain ways to reach an opinion readily come to mind: 1) intuition, 2) imitation, 3) emotion, 4) attraction to an idea, and 5) objective supportive evidence. An opinion that will stand the test of time may be reached by any of these. The history of the search for causes and treatments of illnesses offers many examples of both erroneous and accurate opinions gained by each of these ways. However, in matters of health, opinions supported by objective evidence have gained the reputation of being the most trustworthy and successful. Fanciful schools of opinion about cases of symptoms have come and gone while sound opinions supported by facts continue to serve as well. The method developed in modern times to gather objective supportive evidence is known as the scientific-method, which consists of objective observations coupled with controlled experiments.

Much that has been written about food allergy is a compilation of opinions not reached by the scientific method and is to be regarded with skepticism. The approach to management of food allergy and the opinions expressed in this book are the products of scientific study of children suspected of food allergy.

Some of the most enthusiastic followers of the tradition established by Richet, Jr., and Rowe have excused themselves from the responsibility for securing objective evidence to support their opinions (that multitudinous complaints, especially nervous and behavioral, may be due to allergy to traces of even common foods, like sugar) by claiming they are too busy or lack facilities. They arrogantly leave it to others to test the validity of their opinions while blithely behaving as though the truth is in hand.

THE NATURE OF ILLNESS

In Western culture, disease is commonly thought of as a

disturbance in bodily functions induced by specific agents, like microbes, to be treated by a specific remedy, such as an antibiotic. To escape this narrowness and take into account our entire being, the term *illness* is now used to include the mental discomfort and social consequences of the disruption that may be produced by a disease in all aspects of oneself. In ancient times a person was looked upon as an entity—a harmonious integration of many interdependent functions. Later, to expedite detailed analysis and communication of knowledge, the functions came to be grouped under terms like *body, mind,* and *soul.* In seeking causes and cures of disorders of health, emphasis might be placed on physical, mental, or spiritual disturbances. As relief was sought from ill health, help was offered by healers who concerned themselves chiefly with one of these facets and came to be known as physicians, psychologists, magicians, and clergymen. In a struggle for dominance among healers, the separations become rigid and the soul was relegated to the clergy and the body to physicians. The territory in between has been the scene of a continuing struggle among psychologists, psychiatrists, and magicians/charlatans. Each category of healer has been careless and confused about the appropriate application of their special skills.

That all this is not fatuous philosophy can be realized by considering the direct, practical application to clearing the atmosphere of controversy and confusion that has enveloped food allergy. Those allergists who formulate their opinions and conduct their practices in accordance with the scientific method take pains to distinguish physical from psychological origins of symptoms. They are skeptical of theories and treatments advocated by those who depend on their clinical impressions, with the well-known limitations. Scientific physicians are naturally concerned when diagnoses and treatments are based on inadequate evaluation of the origins of symptoms. Unchecked by the restraints of the scientific approach, some healers, cloaked in the language and credentials of physicians, misuse current knowledge of allergy and exploit the needs of ill people whose complaints of various origins are lumped together under food allergy. The controversy is not over different interpretations of sound knowledge but whether the scientific approach to bodily disorders shall prevail and if each category of healer shall ply their expertise appropriately.

IN CONCLUSION

A reader could not be blamed for impatiently skipping these introductory remarks in his haste to get to the main body of this primer. He may lose something if he does. The concepts touched upon are crucial in the development of the approach set forth in the following pages. An understanding of why food allergy has been so often referred to as controversial and confusing and why it need not be should clear the way to an effective use of what follows.

—CHARLES D. MAY, M.D.

Introduction

Mrs. Jones came to my office the other day and, sinking into a chair, said, "My son John has food allergy; every time he eats sugar, his behavior is obnoxious." The purpose of this primer is to help you think critically about this statement, the words used, and their implication. There are numerous books and pamphlets that have been written for laymen on the subject of food allergy. Most of the publications designed for nonmedical people are based on the "clinical" experience of the authors. This means that generally they are composed of observations and anecdotal reports accumulated by the person writing the book; they are not ordinarily based on scientific studies using objective methods to evaluate the reported histories. This book is designed to take a different approach. The principles described here are derived from basic immunologic studies that have been undertaken in the last twenty or so years. The data and results of evaluations discussed are based on objective studies using the *scientific method*, unless otherwise noted. Use of the scientific method means that the evaluation was performed to eliminate the bias of all participants. Using this technique, one can derive information that should eliminate "beliefs" of both subjects and observers. This is a very important concept and procedure, because the elimination of bias means that the body of information collected should have certain physiological explanations. These can be subjected to analysis in such a way that our factual knowledge about the subject can be advanced.

Conclusions that are not based on the scientific method may be useful insofar as they may sometimes lead to healing. However, they are not helpful when one is interested in cause and effect. Most people, when they are ill, go to the physician in an attempt to feel better. They are not always interested in why illness occurs, but they are usually interested in feeling better.

Healing comes in many different disguises. Most of us would agree that the "snake oil" from the back of patent medicine wagons in the nineteenth-century western United States wasn't very effective nor at times very safe. Yet many people undoubtedly benefited from swallowing these foul potions. Usually, the peddler didn't wait around to survey the results of his treatments, but sold as much as he could and hastily departed to the next town.

Shamans of many varieties have been around as long as man has organized in groups and persist today in many cultures. Some of their herbs probably have specific physiological benefits, and certainly their incantations are very powerful. I once saw a young lady in the hospital who was paralyzed from the waist down. After consultations by many very knowledgeable physicians in a university hosptial, everyone was quite certain that this was a hysterical paralysis or, in medical jargon, a "conversion reaction." Unfortunately, none of the usual approaches to this problem seemed to help. When a "healer" from her ethnic background was finally called in to perform his magic, he had this little girl out of bed and walking in two days. We must never underestimate the power of our beliefs to influence our health.

Healing by means other than scientific medicine may have its place, but it is inappropriate to base regulatory or public health decisions upon information using empirical rather than scientific data gathering procedures. Furthermore, expensive procedures or evaluations that are not based on sound data increase the cost of health care for everyone.

Throughout the history of mankind and his technology, the scientific method has been the tried and true means by which we have reached the advanced level of comfort that we enjoy in our society. There have been long periods of darkness and antiintellectualism, but over the eons these have subsequently been replaced by a return to rational thinking, giving rise to startling advances in our understanding to improve our quality of life.

It is appropriate to question things that we encounter in our environment and to ask searching questions about their effect on us. However, it is also appropriate to answer those questions by collecting information using an objective, nonimpassioned approach.

A number of areas under the general heading of food allergy are discussed in this primer. The first chapter is a consideration of basic principles and definitions that should aid in the understanding of subsequent chapters. Chapter 2 discusses the symptoms and foods that are problems. The information contained in the chapter on skin testing is meant to be a general consideration of this procedure in addition to the specific discussion of skin testing for foods, and chapter 4 discusses other diagnostic tests that are available.

The following chapters contain the approach to confirmation of adverse reactions, the treatment, and the prognosis. In the chapter on controversial procedures, the author's opinions as well as those of other people are stated clearly. Illustrative case histories are included to clarify some points discussed. Finally, a glossary is included to aid in understanding of frequently used terms, and the bibliography will enable interested readers to delve further into the subject.

This primer is designed to be clear about the current facts and myths in this field. Some effort may be required on the part of the reader, because many of the concepts presented here do not usually reach the lay press. It is hoped that the primer will aid the reader's own critical thinking in any area between general information and the complexities of the medical literature.

Food Allergy

I

Basic Principles and Definitions

If one is to understand the way in which adverse reactions to foods occur, it is important to grasp a few basic biological principles. First is the fact that there are a number of possible causes for adverse reactions to foods aside from allergy. Therefore, when we associate some type of symptoms with ingestion of a food, it is important to think of these as adverse reactions rather than allergy. Probably the most common adverse reaction to a food is due to a deficiency in the intestinal enzyme lactase. Lactase digests the milk sugar, lactose, into its two component sugars, which may then be absorbed through the gastrointestinal surface (mucosa). If the enzyme is present in less than normal quantities (which is usually the case, as opposed to complete absence), then the lactose acts as a laxative. There are other enzyme deficiencies that may occur in small children and are responsible for adverse reactions to food.

A second cause of adverse reactions to foods is toxic substances in foods. These may be noxious natural constituents such as alkaloids in mushrooms, cyanide in the stones of some fruit, or many others. (See table.) There are also toxins that contaminate food such as mercury or aflatoxins, which are very toxic substances produced by molds that may contaminate corn or peanuts.

Psychological reactions are commonly the basis for eliminating foods from the diet of many people. Beliefs about what a food will do to someone are very strongly held, and it is difficult to dissuade any one from such beliefs. The manner in which these beliefs are derived is a fascinating subject for both research and speculation. It is also extraordinarily entertaining at times. Every

POTENTIALLY NOXIOUS SUBSTANCES IN FOODSTUFFS

Natural Constituents

Alkaloids (as in mushrooms)
Hemagglutinins (as in beans)
Goitrogens (as in cabbage)
Pressor Amines (as in bananas)
Oxalates (as in rhubarb)
Many unknown

Contaminants

Saxitoxins (from parasite of shrimp)
Ergot
Aflatoxins (from fungus in peanuts, grains)
Penicillin
Mercury
Pesticides

reader will recall amusing stories overheard at social gatherings where people described rather dramatic examples of "food allergy." Our observations support the notion that many of these beliefs have come about because of coincidences, some of which are explained in this book.

This primer is devoted to allergic or sensitivity reactions. Understanding of some basic biological terms is essential in order to comprehend the mechanisms by which foods have been shown to interact with the immune system.

The immune system is the collection of organs, cells, and molecules that are responsible for both protective and adverse responses to substances encountered in the environment.

Antigens are molecules, usually proteins, that have the property of stimulating the immune system to produce a response. *Antiodies* are molecules formed by the body (the immune system) as a very specific response to antigens. The antibodies may be found in the circulation, attached to cells in various parts of the body, and on body surfaces. When antibodies are present (as detected by multiple methods), then the patient may be said to be sensitized.

Immunoglobulin is the specific term used to refer to molecules of antibody. There are five classes of immunoglobulin, at least two of which are important in adverse reactions to foods related to the immune system. These two classes of immunoglobulin (antibody) are called Immunoglobulin G (IgG) and Immunoglobulin E (IgE). IgG is found in the circulatory system and can attach to antigens and aid in their elimination and thus may be protective. In certain circumstances, the IgG may combine with the antigen and then interact with certain cells or other molecules produced in the body to cause damage to other cells.

Immunoglobulin E is the principal antibody associated with "allergic" reactions, as the term *allergy* is often used in lay literature. The important characteristic of IgE is that it binds to cells called *MAST* cells. These cells contain small chemicals called mediators, which can cause various types of reactions in the body. One of these mediators is called histamine. When histamine is injected into the skin (or when it is released by the body's own cells), it causes wheal and flare reactions commonly known as urticaria or hives. This skin reaction is often called a welt. Itching is probably produced by the stimulation of nerve fibers responsible for the sensation of itching. Each year numerous new biochemicals that are part of immune reactions are identified. As the list grows ever longer, it becomes clear that many symptoms are due to multiple biochemical reactions, making treatment more complicated.

The term *allergy* is confusing, especially when applied to the topic of foods, because it has two components: symptoms and sensitization (presence of antibodies). When someone reports to me that he/she has a food allergy, he/she is usually describing symptoms. But the term *allergy* refers to the presence of antibodies as well as symptoms. Because this term has been misused and confused, we have adopted other terms that use both components—symptoms and sensitization.

Symptomatic food sensitivity is present when the patient has antibodies detected by one or another laboratory method and when a double-blind food challenge (as described below) demonstrates the presence of symptoms. It is also assumed that other causes of adverse reactions to foods have been eliminated as possibilities. In this situation, the patient has *symptoms* and *antibodies* and, therefore, has *symptomatic sensitivity*.

When the patient has detectable antibodies but no symptoms occur when the food is ingested, then the patient has *asymptomatic sensitivity*. The latter situation confuses people, because a subject can have one or more positive skin tests to foods that are eaten without causing any symptoms. This should not be referred to as a false positive test, nor is the skin test incorrect. (*False positive* means something that seems to happen for one particular reason but is actually happening for an unrelated reason.) If the skin test is done properly, the patient does have the antibodies, but when the food protein is eaten, not enough protein gets to the antibodies to produce a reaction. Another way to think about this is that if the same food protein were given to the patient intravenously, thus avoiding the body's natural barriers, it would often cause a severe reaction (anaphylaxis) and thus prove that the antibodies detected are significant.

These terms apply to things we inhale as well as foods we eat. Many people have been tested by allergists and found to have positive skin tests to animal dander, yet they live with animals and have *no* symptoms. This too is asymptomatic sensitivity.

People wonder why they have allergic symptoms. The ability to respond adversely to things in the environment occurs in families and is controlled by our genes. In addition to foods, people have allergic reactions to things they inhale (pollen, animal dander) and to things that are injected (medication, insect venom). Everyone with a normal immune system probably has the capacity to have an allergic reaction. Exactly why some people have such severe problems while others have no problems is not known at this time. The initiating factors—that is, why the problem begins in some people at six months of age, some at six years of age, and some in adulthood—is also unclear. In children there is often a sequence of symptoms beginning in infancy with diarrhea and eczema and progressing to asthma and allergic rhinitis (hay fever). Most children are only afflicted with one of these problems in their early years, and often the problem is transient.

II

Reported Symptoms and Incriminated Foods

REPORTED SYMPTOMS

Symptoms attributed to adverse reactions to foods fall into four major groups and some minor ones.

Gastrointestinal Reactions

Symptoms related to the gastrointestinal tract are nausea, abdominal pains, vomiting, and diarrhea. These are the most commonly reported of all symptoms due to adverse reactions to foods and the most commonly confirmed by proper testing. Some of these reactions to foods are obvious and very impressive. Patients who eat nuts may have the immediate onset of nausea, vomiting, and marked abdominal pain. Less obvious is chronic diarrhea in children, which may be produced by a number of foods, the most common of which appear to be milk, soy, and wheat.

Colic in infants caused by food ingestion, especially milk ingestion, by either the child or the nursing mother is currently under investigation. The symptoms of colic in infants include irritability, chronic crying, drawing up of the legs thought to be caused by cramps, and difficulty sleeping. A minority of children studied thus far have improved when one or more foods were removed from the mother's or child's diet. Since these children are rather difficult to live with, a brief elmination diet may be justified. When asked about colic, I reply that if one of these "screamers" lived in my house, we'd try an elimination diet. If it helped, we'd put the food back in the diet and see if the symptoms returned. Often they do not. If they do, the food may usually be reintroduced at one-month intervals until the symptoms no longer occur. This is because the problem is quickly outgrown in the vast majority of infants.

Skin Symptoms

Two major types of skin rashes have been associated with food ingestion. The most commonly seen and agreed upon as being caused by food allergy are urticaria (hives, often referred to by patients as welts). These are usually red raised bumps, which may have a white center. They are usually very itchy. Any area of the body may be involved, but the palms and soles are usually spared.

Swelling of the lips, ears, eyes, face, and occasionally other areas of the body is called angioedema. Angioedema is similar to hives but occurs deeper in the skin. The chemistry of both these reactions is similar to that of a positive skin test, as explained in the chapter on skin testing.

Eczema (atopic dermatitis) is the second type of skin rash frequently associated with food allergy. It is a very itchy, scaly skin rash, which in infants appears as small bumps, usually white or red, over the face and neck. As children get older, persistent eczema localizes to the inner surface of the arm, opposite the elbows, and behind the knees. Dermatologists and allergists have disagreed about the allergic nature of eczema. In the last few years, clear evidence from objective challenges has shown that some children's eczema is aggravated by eating certain foods. Most children with eczema do not have food allergy. In those that do, foods are only part of the problem, and it is rare to see eczema completely disappear using elimination diets. As with the youngsters with colic, a one-week elimination diet in children with eczema is easy to perform, inexpensive, often helpful, and only temporarily aggravating to the children.

Other skin rashes, including generalized redness, facial flushing, and diaper rashes, seem to be related to ingestion of some fruits and vegetables. Oranges and tomatoes produce these reactions in young children, but the responsible mechanism is unclear. The immune system has not been shown to play a role in these reactions, so they should not be called allergy.

Respiratory Symptoms

Persistent runny or stuffy nose (nasal congstion), especially in the first three years of life, is often blamed on food allergy, particularly milk allergy. When milk or other foods are removed from the diet, the problem often seems better. Since the condition is usually transient anyway, the reintroduction of food into the diet often is not accompanied by a return of the problem. In fact, it is quite difficult to prove an association between chronic nasal symptoms and food ingestion. Thus this is another symptom that should not be called allergic unless the food and the symptom can be clearly related and it can be proven that the immune system is involved.

Asthma, wheezing, or a chronic cough has been attributed to food allergy, and many children and adults have been subjected to unpleasant dietary restrictions as part of their asthma therapy. However, wheezing or cough as the sole manifestation of food allergy is rather uncommon in controlled studies using objective food challenges in asthma sufferers. Asthmatics who suffer enough from their illness should not be subjected to prolonged dietary elimination without substantial proof of benefit.

Perhaps the most controversial and difficult problem is chronic or recurrent ear infections in preschool children. Many children with this problem are subjected to an elimination diet, most often a dairy-product–free diet, without much evidence of benefit. Often the ear infections continue despite the diet and the milk exclusion becomes prolonged. Ear infections are a difficult problem because they could have a permanent effect on hearing and if they do not respond to treatment, surgery to place polyethylene tubes in the eardrum is often necessary. These reasons are often used as justification for prolonged elimination diets.

In view of the lack of proof that food allergy causes ear infections, I am skeptical at this time about the usefulness of a prolonged elimination diet, which is usually unpleasant for the entire family. If the ear infections are not a problem during the summer months, which is usually the case, it seems unlikely that any food in the diet is responsible for the problem. In those children with infections, even during the summer, consideration of dietary therapy may be warranted, but not for a prolonged period. We still need a definitive way to demonstrate a direct relationship between food ingestion and ear problems in young children. Early studies now underway with infant monkeys may ultimately help us learn more about this problem in infant humans.

In spite of these comments, the possibility remains that allergens, especially inhaled ones, are involved in chronic ear infections. In experimental studies, middle ear changes can be induced by the rather artificial method of spraying pollen into the nose. These studies have been undertaken in adults and not in children and not yet with foods. Children's anatomy may also be a problem, because once the eustachian tube (the tube from the back of the nose to the middle ear) becomes inflamed, the middle ear is like an abscess and only drainage (with polyethylene tubes) will relieve the problem.

Behavioral Changes

Children's behavior is by far the symptom most intertwined with diet by laymen. Hyperactivity, attention problems, fatigue, anxiety, and numerous other behavioral symptoms have been blamed on every possible dietary constituent, including sugar, dyes, additives, and preservatives. Hyperactivity has received the most attention because of reported dramatic "cures" on various elimination diets. Whole books have been written on this subject and have achieved such popularity that there are parents' groups that promote the idea. The reader should be aware that the overwhelming number of these claims that so permeate the lay literature and media talk shows have never been confirmed by proper studies. Those painstaking studies that have been carried out have rarely confirmed the reported behavioral changes, making it unlikely that millions of children throughout the world are afflicted with the problem. The reason for the impressive claims seems to be related to the power of positive thinking, which persuades people that dietary changes will make them feel better. This may be viewed as laudable by some people, but it may also be seen as an unnecessary crutch that may provoke a new set of problems if the child sees himself or herself as different or ill. Dietary restrictions are also seen by children as punishment for things over which they may have no control.

Two groups of children seem to be subjected to dietary changes for their behavior. One group are those children who are truly different behaviorally than their peers, who may have trouble succeeding in school, and who are a trial to their parents, teachers, and themselves. One can certainly sympathize with the desire to find an easy solution to this complex problem.

The second group are normal children who are supposed to behave differently only when given certain foods or constituents of food. These children are the easiest to study because the behavior due to the suspected food is so different from their normal disposition. Our studies of this type of child have yet to confirm any behavioral changes when the child and observers do not know when the child is getting the incriminated food.

I suspect that an observation about behavioral change occurs in a setting that might excite any child and then the change is blamed on a food. The behavior is perpetuated because everyone expects that when the child receives that food a problem will occur. The power of suggestion is certainly strong enough to produce such a result.

Fortunately, quality behavioral research is continuing. Although it takes time, it will certainly lead to proper answers one day. In the meantime, I strongly urge parents to view the association between behavioral changes and foods with a very critical eye. Chapter 6 offers a simple method by which some observations can be tested at home.

Other Symptoms Attributed to Food

Arthritis has been ascribed to food allergy, and dramatic cures have been credited to elimination diets. Similar claims have been made about recurrent urinary tract infections, Meniere's disease (a problem of the inner ear), and many types of headaches. Despite numerous testimonials concerning these and other problems, the reader is advised to carefully consider any recommendations about undergoing expensive and dislocating dietary evaluation and therapy. A second opinion is often advisable and helps by providing a critical perspective about the problem and recommended treatments.

Migraine headaches have recently been subjected to careful study with elimination diets and double-blind food challenges. The results must be considered preliminary, but some patients appear to have truly benefited by removal of certain foods from their diets. The foods seem to have been triggering the headaches in some cases although whether these reactions are allergy is not yet certain. We must be clear about the fact that many people claim benefit for their headaches but have not separated real benefit from the placebo effect of confirming a strongly held belief. The patients referred to in this paragraph have had their headaches triggered even when their bias has been eliminated by blind food challenge.

Incriminated Foods

Every food, additive, preservative, and dye has been blamed for some type of adverse reactions. Restricting oneself to those foods, confirmed by properly performed food challenges (see chapter 5), vastly shortens the list. By far the most common offenders are nuts. These include peanuts, which are actually legumes, or members of the bean family, including soy, peas, lentils, lima beans, and others. Fish and shellfish are also fairly common offenders. Eggs and milk account for a large number of reactions. Many other foods have been confirmed in a few cases.

It is surprising how infrequently "food villains" have been proven to cause adverse reactions. Probably the number one culprit is chocolate. While there have been a few cases of confirmed reactions to chocolate during blind food challenges, we are still looking for our first after evaluating hundreds of patients for food allergy. Other villains that have been infrequently proved to cause a reaction are strawberries, grains (especially corn), sugar, and citrus fruits. As noted earlier, fruits do seem to cause a facial flush and diaper rash in some small children, but we have not been able to show that this reaction is related to the immune system, and these reactions are quickly outgrown.

It was found during very careful studies of very allergic peanut and soy subjects that they do not react to the purified oils of these foods (e.g. peanut and soy oils).

Timing of Reactions

Adverse reactions to foods are said to be either immediate or delayed. The former occur in minutes to an hour or two, while the latter are said to occur hours to days after the food is eaten. Some claims are made that the food must be eaten several times a day or several days in succession in order to produce symptoms.

Food challenge studies have proven the existence and characteristics of the reaction occurring in minutes to hours. Diarrhea in small children has been the major reaction occurring days after foods are eaten. Most of the delayed reactions attributed to foods are subjective symptoms that have been triggered during open elimination and dietary challenges.

Continuing research is needed to define the spectrum of foods, symptoms, and timing of reactions. This can only be properly performed using blind food challenges. As time passes we hope to discover better diagnostic tests to help in our fundamental understanding of these issues. Chapter 5 considers specific clinical examples of some of the points made in this chapter.

III

Skin Testing

Skin tests may be used to diagnose food allergy just as they are used to diagnose allergy to environmental inhalants (substances in the air that are inhaled). Skin tests are used to detect antibodies of a certain type (IgE as described above), which indicate that a person has the potential to react to the substance. It must be emphasized that for foods *or* inhalants a positive skin test only means that antibodies are present and, therefore, the potential to react is present. There is not an absolute (100 percent) correlation between the presence of a positive skin test and the presence of symptoms. The correlation is made by a thorough history and sometimes appropriate challenge tests. If confusion is to be avoided, the point must be vigorously stressed that skin tests do not make a diagnosis; they only measure probability.

SKIN TEST EXTRACTS

Skin test materials for both foods and inhalants are prepared by making an extract of the substances to be used. Extraction means collection of a fraction (usually a mixture of proteins) of the substance into a solution that can be sterilized and safely applied to the skin. These extracts are usally prepared by commercial manufacturers.

Before they are used, the contents of extracts for skin testing should be verified. Verification means that they are shown not to be irritants in the skin of normal people and that they do detect specific antibodies in the people who have those antibodies. If enough of any material is injected into the skin, a red bump will be formed. Therefore, if the test is not performed carefully and with proper dilutions, anyone can be made to have a positive skin test.

TECHNIQUES OF SKIN TESTING

Below are described the methods of skin testing shown by the scientific method to be reliable. Puncture or prick skin tests are performed by placing a drop of extract on the patient's back or arm and making a small dent in the skin with a needle. The skin may also be lightly tented to achieve the same effect. A scratch test is performed by making a small scratch (usually about 5 mm) in the skin and then placing a drop of extract over the scratch. The intradermal test is performed by using a very small needle, which is placed just into the skin, and a very small amount of material (less than 0.1 cc) is injected into the skin. This test will remind readers of a TB (tuberculosis) skin test but involves injecting less material.

The goal of each of these techniques is to inject a small amount of material into the skin for the detection of antibody. The puncture test injects the smallest amount of material into the skin, thus requiring that the patient have a fairly large amount of antibody in order to respond. The intradermal test injects material farther into the skin, thus requiring that the patient have less antibody in order to respond.

After about twenty minutes, the skin is examined for the presence of a wheal and flare (hive) at the site of each test. The presence of a hive means that there is antibody present and that it has caused the release of chemicals called mediators. One of these mediators is histamine, and it causes the formation of a hive by causing fluid (plasma) to leak from small blood vessels.

Skin tests are measured in a number of different ways. At times there seem to be as many ways to score the test as there are people doing the scoring. The most important part is the wheal, the raised portion. In my opinion (the minority), the easiest thing to do is measure the approximate diameter of the wheal (the bump) and ignore the flare, which may be quite large or small and is irrelevant. Most allergists use a system of pluses; for example, 1+ may be a flare with no wheal while 4+ may be a large wheal surrounded by small ones. Since there is no standardization, the pluses may mean different things to different allergists. The most important part of skin testing is not the wording of the size of the test but rather interpretation of the results.

Intradermal skin tests are often used when a skin reaction is not found but the doctor strongly suspects the patient is reacting to a particular substance. In my opinion, intradermal skin tests for foods should be used rarely. Intradermal skin tests for foods or inhalant substances should never be done in large numbers because they are more likely than prick/puncture tests to yield information not related to the patient's symptoms. In other words, the test may be positive but symptoms don't occur when the food is eaten or the patient has asymptomatic sensitivity (chapter 1).

Research studies have shown that for skin testing with extracts of inhalants (pollens, molds, danders) there is an approximate association between the size of the wheal produced and the probability that a reaction will occur when the patient is exposed to the substance in a controlled challenge. The bigger the skin reaction, the more likely that symptoms will occur. For foods this has not been found to be true. A small skin reaction may be associated with a pronounced symptomatic response, and a large skin reaction may not be accompanied by any symptoms when the food is consumed.

The confusion occurs when a person is skin tested to many foods and has numerous positive responses. The person receives a list of foods and is told that he is allergic to these and they should be avoided. Usually the patient has been consuming many of these foods without problems and then is puzzled as to the meaning of the test. The way to solve this dilemma is by food challenges, as discussed in chapter 5.

Skin testing in young children is often said to be worthless. In fact, skin testing in children of any age (including infants) may be extremely helpful if properly performed and interpreted. The procedure is not terribly uncomfortable, and most youngsters cry only because they are made to hold still. Recently it has been found that the skin tests may be placed on the back (or arm) and then wiped off and the child may be allowed to play during the fifteen to twenty minutes required for the reaction to appear. This procedure limits the ''holding-still time'' to a few minutes and diminishes youthful protests. Young children should be skin tested for foods (or inhalants) that are suspected of producing symptoms rather than with an arbitrary battery of tests. Positive skin tests indicate that the child *may* have symptoms related to ingestion of the food, but this must be confirmed by food challenge.

IV

Other Diagnostic Tests

There are numerous diagnostic tests that have been employed for the evaluation of patients with food sensitivity. Those that will be considered in this section are those that have been shown to have some validity, whereas other tests that are used but have not been shown to be helpful are considered in a later section.

RADIOALLERGOSORBENT TEST (RAST)

The RAST test is a biochemical assay that detects the antibodies similar to those detected by skin tests and is performed on blood samples rather than on the skin. This test requires the use of radiation, but because it is done in a laboratory, there is no direct contact between the patient and the radiation. The test has been shown to be no more useful than skin tests for detecting the antibodies that allergists are seeking. The RAST has some particular problems in interpretation, and results of the test are often misinterpreted. It is an excellent research tool but should only be used in very special clinical situations, where it may be a helpful diagnostic test. Because of the hazards of radiation and the problems with disposal, this test is being replaced by an enzyme test. However, this too has not yet been shown to be any more useful than a skin test.

Recently, the RAST has been touted by numerous people, many not allergists or even physicians, as the answer to allergy diagnosis. There are places in the country where the test can be obtained without being ordered by a physician. Treatment by unqualified people is then prescribed based on the test results.

I cannot *stress too strongly* that thousands of people are spending millions of dollars for testing that is unnecessary, improperly performed, and incorrectly interpreted and serves as a basis for treatment recommendations that may be totally invalid. This is especially true for food allergy, where a positive test is often used as the reason to eliminate foods from the diet.

In view of the very high cost of the test compared to skin testing and the fact that no more information is acquired than with properly performed skin tests, patients would be wise to question their physician closely about the need for this test, should it be suggested. This opinion is in accord with the 1983 American Academy of Allergy and Immunology's position paper on RAST testing.

MEASUREMENT OF SPECIFIC SERUM ANTIBODIES

There are a number of techniques available for measuring antibodies in the serum that have been formed against specific food proteins. These antibodies are helpful in enabling the physician to determine whether or not an individual has more antibody to certain food proteins than other people of the same age. This test does not directly diagnose an adverse reaction, but, rather, it tells the physician that the food in question should be examined carefully as a possible offending food. At the present time this test is not available in many places. However, in the future its availability should be increasing.

An antibody that is commonly measured is the *total* IgE antibody. This test should not be confused with the RAST (discussed above), which measures *specific* IgE antibody. The *total* IgE antibody may be increased in patients with allergy to food or inhalants, but it may be normal. Conversely, the patient may have allergy, but the total IgE may be normal. Thus this test alone cannot be used to make a diagnosis of allergy. It is arguable whether or not it is even a good screening test. In my opinion, when skin testing is available, that is the preferred test.

BIOPSY OF THE MUCOSA OF THE SMALL INTESTINE

It is often not realized that chronic diarrhea may be the product of an adverse reaction to a food. This reaction is produced because an alteration in the normal surface (mucosa) of the small intestine is produced by an interaction between the food and something in the intestine. At the present time, there is considerable evidence supporting the theory that this interaction occurs between the food and the immune system, which then produces the abnormal intestinal surface. When this occurs, ingested nutrients are not well absorbed and the patient tends to develop diarrhea. For one food in particular, wheat gluten, the food protein may produce a very severe abnormality in the intestinal surface. When this occurs, the only definitive diagnostic test is a biopsy of the small intestine. This is accomplished by passing a small tube, which has a capsule on the end, into the small intestine and taking a small piece of tissue, which may then be examined under the microscope and also used for various laboratory measurements. Because of the severe nature of celiac disease, or gluten-sensitive enteopathy, it is imperative that the biopsy test be used so that the diagnosis may be made unequivocally. This appears to be a lifelong illness, and for most patients it is necessary to exclude wheat gluten from the diet permanently. In small children, two other proteins that produce a similar but transient condition are milk protein and soy protein. The abnormality produced by these proteins usually resolves by the third birthday. There are other foods that have been incriminated in the production of this reaction, but at the present time, these observations require further confirmation.

BLOOD COUNTS

Often patients will have a white blood cell count done and then be told they have allergy. This happens because there are cells in the blood (also in the nasal mucus, the airway to the lungs, and the intestine), which are called eosinophils. It is true that these cells may be present when allergic reactions occur, but there are also many other reasons for their presence. Therefore, sometimes there may be increased numbers of eosinophils present in the blood but the patient will not be found to have detectable allergy.

V

Food Challenges

This chapter is devoted to a discussion of the objective evaluation of patients complaining of an adverse reaction to a food. Studies have shown that *less than half* the impressive histories of adverse reactions to food in children can be confirmed by *objective* food challenges.

In order for a food challenge to be successful, it must be performed in a manner that eliminates the bias of the patient and observers, that reproduces the conditions under which the reaction has been reported to occur, and that allows observation and measurement of the symptoms. Thus the first step in any procedure for evaluating an adverse reaction to a food is to eliminate the symptoms about which the patient is complaining. This is ordinarily accomplished by an elimination diet that may be as simple as removing one food from the diet or as complex as placing the patient on a completely elemental liquid diet containing no substances to which the patient could react. When the subject's symptoms have been eliminated for a period of time so that any normal variation of the symptoms is understood, then it is appropriate to perform the food challenge. Food challenges are properly performed by administering the food in question in a double-blind manner. The term *double-blind* means that the food is administered so that neither the subject nor the persons responsible for making the observations know what the subject is receiving. At times, it is necessary to use a placebo when food challenges are being performed.

A placebo is a substance that is not known to have any physiological effect on the body, but to which psychological responses occur as often as one-third of the time. Using a placebo allows the objective administraton of one challenge to which the subject should not have any symptoms. If the subject has a reaction to a placebo, then one may be certain that the reaction is not due to the suspected food. A few additional comments about the placebo effect are important. In pharmaceutical and other studies that use placebos, it is usually observed that about one-third or more of the subjects report significant improvement in their symptoms while receiving the placebo treatment. There are examples of very impressive symptoms: severe chest pain, headaches, and even measurable physiological changes being altered by placebo treatment. Thus a patient may appear to have an impressive physiological response to a substance that itself has no physiological effect. These responses are presumably controlled by the patient's brain and nervous system. We should never underestimate the power of the human brain to heal or to deceive the body.

The best way to perform a double-blind food challenge is to use opaque capsules and to administer the food in small but increasing amounts over the period of time that the patient has reported will be required to reproduce the symptoms. The capsules are prepared by using powdered foods, which are available for many substances. The dried foods are placed in capsules and then the capsules administered to the patient. Obviously, for small children and in certain exceptional situations capsules cannot be used. In small children, however, it is easy to hide or disguise many foods in either formula, apple sauce, or something that the child is usually eating. The food challenges are best administered in the physician's office, where systematic observations can be made and recorded. In some instances it may be necessary to send the subject home with several days' supply of food capsules, which are taken on a prescribed schedule. In this situation, the patient may have two sets of capsules: one that will be the active food and one that will be the placebo. It is clearly imperative for the patient to be willing to remain uninformed about the contents of the capsules.

It is very important that both the patient and the physician have a strong desire to ascertain the correct answer rather than to confirm either of their beliefs. If a patient has a strongly held belief that a certain food will cause a certain reaction and the patient is unwilling to even consider the possibility that this may be incorrect, it is futile to perform a food challenge and the patient should be left to cope with the belief in whatever way seems comfortable. The major purpose of food challenges is to determine in an objective, unbiased manner whether or not an adverse reaction is truly related to the ingestion of a food.

Careful studies have been shown that in children from a few months to sixteen years of age, approximately 60 percent of the impressive histories of adverse reaction cannot be confirmed when a double-blind food challenge is administered. This means that, for whatever reason, the patient acquired a belief about an adverse reaction that was thought to occur when a food was ingested, but that this reaction does not occur due to physiological processes.

EXAMPLES OF DOUBLE-BLIND FOOD CHALLENGES

Susie, a seven-year-old girl, had a history of marked urticaria (hives) followed by the onset of wheezing within one or two hours after eating one or two peanuts or one-fourth of a peanut butter sandwich. This child also had a history of severe asthma, which required frequent hospitalizations and evaluation at a residential treatment center for asthmatic children. She had a markedly positive skin test to peanuts. When Susie was challenged with peanut in capsules in slowly increasing amounts, the urticarial reaction in the skin was produced within fifteen minutes of the time she ingested the peanuts. She did not, however, experience the subsequent onset of wheezing. This challenge was attempted on three occasions in order to try to reproduce the asthma symptoms, but wheezing did not occur. She also did not have any gastrointestinal complaints.

Comments: It was possible to reproduce the skin symptoms but not the respiratory ones. In reviewing the history of the wheezing episodes, which had previously been associated with eating peanuts, the patient and her mother reported that she became markedly upset and agitated on the occasions when she had broken out with urticaria. It is quite possible, and has frequently been seen, that situations that are upsetting for children with marked asthma can produce the onset of wheezing. Although it is possible for children (and adults) to wheeze when eating peanuts, the only symptom that could be reproduced in Susie was the skin symptom.

Johnny was a ten-month-old who had been breast-fed exclusively until approximately eight months of age. At that time, cow milk had been introduced into his diet, and he had begun to exhibit, within two to three weeks, an increase in spitting, which had previously been noted, apparent cramps, characterized by crying and drawing up of his legs within hours after eating, and much looser stools, which were occasionally very watery and ran out of his diapers. Solid foods, which had previously been introduced into the diet, were removed, but the gastrointestinal symptoms continued. When Johnny was placed on an elemental formula, his symptoms—including frequent spitting—completely disappeared. He was subsequently challenged by placing small but increasing amounts of cow milk formula in the elemental formula, and it was discovered that when he received two ounces at a single feeding, his gastrointestinal symptoms were reproduced. Reviewing the history with the mother elicited the information that during the time that she was nursing Johnny, if she consumed more than sixteen ounces per day of milk or had what she termed a "dairy product binge" that included cheese, ice cream, and milk, he would be more fussy and his spitting would seem to increase. She had previously not associated these dietary excesses with his symptoms. When Johnny was skin tested with an extract of cow milk, he was noted to have a small but definitely positive skin test reaction.

Johnny was challenged at monthly intervals after the diagnosis was made. The challenges began with an amount smaller than that which produced the previous reaction and was increased until symptoms began to appear. Over four months, the tolerated amounts increased until, at about fourteen months, milk was tolerated in the diet.

Comments: It should be noted, as discussed under skin testing, that skin testing may be extremely helpful in youngsters like Johnny, when it is positive. If the skin test is negative, it does not absolutely eliminate the possibility of the particular food being a problem. However, the probability that the antibodies (IgE) detected by skin testing are responsible for the symptoms is very unlikely. When the skin test is positive, it indicates that the food may be a problem and that the immune system (IgE) is involved in producing the symptom. (The reader is reminded to review the terms *symptomatic* and *asymptomatic sensitivity*.) Adverse reactions in babies following nursing to foods in the diet of their mother are not common, but definitely occur. If the mother's diet is not examined and altered systematically with regard for her nutrition and that of the baby, both may have a nutritionally inadequate diet. I have seen instances when enough foods have been removed from the mother's diet to produce malnutrition in the baby. In these cases, the mother needs nutritional, as well as medical, assistance to provide her with a nutritionally adequate diet. Occasionally, these children must be weaned. Although this is rare, it does occur, and it is deplorable that sometimes mothers are made to feel guilty because of the confusion surrounding the proper diagnosis.

Repeated challenges using small amounts of milk showed that Johnny's reaction was "outgrown" over the next four months. The physiological basis of this loss of reaction is not understood at this time.

Billy was a six-year-old who was referred with a reported

history that eating a doughnut for breakfast made him a "monster" the rest of the day. This had been going on for approximatly one year; whenever he had doughnuts for breakfast, there were significant complaints about uncontrollable behavior from both his mother when he spent the day at home and from his schoolteacher if he was at school. When we were reviewing the onset of this history with Billy's mother, she could not quite recall how she had arrived at the association between food and behavior, but it had become extrapolated from doughnuts to sugar in general. She was certain that any time Billy received any significant quantities of sugar, as small an amount as might be contained in one piece of hard candy, his behavior would become uncontrollable.

Billy was a delightful young man who was a pleasure to be around. A scoring system was designed that would evaluate his behavior, and, because he was very cooperative, it was possible to use capsules containing sugar to do the double-blind challenge. Billy was given double the amount of sugar that was calculated to be in a single doughnut three times a day for one week. The challenge was designed to take four weeks. During this time, he got sugar three times a day every day for one week, a placebo consisting of a food that he clearly tolerated three times a day every day for a second week, and then sugar again, and, finally, placebo again. During this time, there was neither alteration in his behavior nor did he exhibit the hyperactive or disconcerting behavior. At the end of this challenge, the process was explained to Billy and his reward was to be given a doughnut for dessert after each meal for three days. He was told that we had not been able to change his behavior with the sugar-containing capsules and that, therefore, we were certain that he would not react when he ate the doughnut and this was his reward. In fact, when he was given the open challenge, we were unable to reproduce any behavioral alterations described by this mother. A six-month and one-year conversation with Billy and his mother revealed that he was not having any unusual problems with his behavior.

Comments: Billy is one example of several behavioral problems in children that we have evaluated. We have as yet been unable to reproduce the behavioral alterations associated with the ingestion of sugar when a double-blind challenge is performed. There is a great deal of misinformation and innuendo in the lay press concerning sugar and food additive ingestion, and while there may be an occasional patient who really does have some kind of problem with sugar ingestion producing behavioral symptoms, we have been unable to reproduce this reaction. We have seen children who are truly hyperactive but in whom dietary manipulations have made no significant change in the behavior. This particular subject is emotionally charged amongst laymen and the medical profession. Careful, dispassionate analysis using objective methods including blind challenges are required to finally settle the matter. (See chapter 6 for suggested techniques to examine this problem at home.)

Sylvia was a forty-five-old nurse with a reported history of arthritis, which began approximately two years prior to her initial visit. In the preceding six months, she had become concerned about the possible association between ingestion of wheat and perhaps other foods, but most particularly wheat, and exacerbations of her arthritis. An increase in her arthritis symptoms occurred a couple of times per month, and she felt that when they were associated with wheat ingestion, they had been severe and incapacitating. She felt that in the several weeks prior to her visit when she had avoided wheat, she had been less troubled by her arthritis. We arranged a double-blind food challenge to wheat using capsules, because she reported that the quantity required to induce symptoms was quite small and we were able to place more than this amount in the number of capsules that could conveniently be consumed at one sitting. The study was planned so that she would keep a symptom score dividing the waking hours into two segments. The challenge was performed at home and required four weeks. On Monday, Tuesday, and Wednesday of each week, she received approximately twenty capsules three times a day. Two sets of capsules contained wheat, and two sets of capsules contained the dextrose placebo. At the end of two weeks and at the end of four weeks, the symptom score was reviewed, but the code of the challenge was not broken until the end of four weeks. The week that she had the most significant symptoms with her arthritis turned out to be a placebo week. There was no reproducible association between wheat ingestion and the arthritis symptoms. When this was discussed with Sylvia at the end of the challenge period, she was naturally ambivalent about the results. On the one hand, she was pleased that she no longer had to worry about eating wheat, and on the other hand, she was disappointed to learn that there was not going to be an easy dietary solution to her arthritis problem.

Comments: Sylvia represents an example where a significant problem seemed helped by dietary manipulation, but because of the nuisance of maintaining a wheat-free diet, she wanted to determine whether there was a true cause and effect relationship. Chronic diseases, especially those that interfere significantly with normal daily activities, are subjected to many dietary manipulations. The lay literature reports startling and fabulous cures of various severe ailments by dietary manipulation. The food challenges are always performed openly, subjecting the observations to the patient's and observer's biases. Although people may feel better while on these diets, the improvement should be viewed as due to the benefits of belief in the healing effect rather than proof of cause and effect. The medical profession is frequently accused of being uninterested in dietary relief or of opposing it, yet the accusers seem to feel no compunction to prove by objective procedures that their claims are true.

Harvey was a twelve-year-old asthmatic whose history of wheezing was often associated with food ingestion earlier in the week. The most prominent example was that if he ate as little as one small piece of chocolate on Sunday, by Tuesday or Wednesday he would be wheezing. There was a history of similarly delayed reactions to other foods. Harvey's mother felt strongly that these "delayed" reactions were a significant cause of his asthma. Harvey was less convinced and reported (when away from his mother) that he often cheated on his diet without triggering wheezing. Chocolate was the food he thought most likely to produce his problem.

The challenge was arranged to reproduce the reported circumstances. First, chocolate or placebo was given on a Monday when there were no asthma symptoms, and symptom scores and objective measurements of airway function were recorded for the rest of the week. When this failed to produce asthma, the challenge was repeated so that staring on a Monday and for the following three days, the chocolate or placebo was given three times a day. This also failed to produce wheezing, and chocolate was added openly to Harvey's diet without being a problem. Challenges either openly (because he had been eating the food on the sly without a reaction) or blindly to the other foods eliminated from his diet failed to cause any delayed-onset of wheezing.

Comments: Delayed-onset reactions to foods several days after ingestion are frequently reported. Our efforts with numerous patients have failed to duplicate the reported reactions during blind challenges. This is another area that requires careful examination using objective methods, because of the strongly held beliefs of many patients and some physicians. Suspicion of delayed-onset reactions is one of the circumstances resulting in very limited diets for some patients. Many foods are easily incriminated but not so easily exonerated.

Tommy was a fourteen-year-old who had a history of a severe reaction to peanuts when he was five years of age. The symptoms of this reaction included generalized redness or flushing, hives (urticaria) on his arms, legs, and trunk, wheezing, and a feeling of faintness. At the time the history was acquired, no additional information was available. A skin test was performed and found to be quite large (10 mm in diameter). Tommy reported that his last known exposure to peanuts had occurred when he was in the second grade and he had eaten a cookie that supposedly contained walnuts. After he had a reaction similar to the one that he first had at age five, the family was able to determine that the person making the cookies had run out of walnuts and substituted peanuts in the last few cookies. Tommy had avoided peanuts knowingly but was brought to us because of his and his parents concern that sooner or later he would have an accidental exposure to peanut and his family wanted to know to what degree he was still sensitive. Reluctantly and very carefully, we decided to help the family determine the answer to their question and began with a minute amount of peanut given blindly in capsules. When we got to the equivalent of a half a peanut, Tommy complained of abdominal pain, nausea, and a general feeling of itching. At this time, he did not exhibit wheezing and his skin did not show any visible sign of a rash. We elected to discontinue the challenge at this point, telling Tommy that an accidental exposure would still be hazardous to his health, and we provided him with a syringe that contained epinephrine.

Comments: This young man illustrates a number of important principles. First, that severe adverse reactions to foods— anaphylaxis—can be lifelong. Although some children do outgrow their severe reactions to foods, as illustrated by the next case, challenges of these children *MUST* be undertaken *ONLY* under direct medical supervision in a facility equipped to provide emergency care. This also illustrates Murphy's Law of food allergy, which says: "If there is a youngster in a class who is very allergic to some food, and it is only being served in a small quantity so that most of the children will not eat it, the allergic youngster is the one who will get the food and have a reaction."

Jennifer was eighteen months old at the time we evaluated her. Her history was that at six months she had been weaned and was first given a cow milk formula. The second or third day, she began vomiting after each feeding, and this became more and more profuse and was followed by diarrhea after each feeding and, finally, on about the third or fourth day, she had profuse vomiting, diarrhea, and a generalized rash. She turned very pale and her mother rushed her to the emergency room, where she was found to be somewhat lethargic and was treated with epinephrine and intravenous fluids. Since that time, she had had no intentional exposure to cow milk, but on one occasion had eaten a small piece of cheese that she found on the floor in the kitchen. This ingestion did not produce any reaction, although it made the family most anxious. A skin test to milk was found to be moderately positive (8 mm in diameter). For the reasons given in the previous case, we elected to undertake a very careful challenge of Jennifer with cow milk. Beginning with a very small amount and increasing very slowly over several days while she remained in the hospital under observation, we did not demonstrate any significant reaction to milk. When she was able to drink six ounces of cow milk and eat a piece of cheese, she complained that her "tummy hurt" and she had some red spots on her face.

Comments: In contrast to Tommy (the previous case), Jennifer was apparently fortunate to outgrow her severe adverse reaction to food. We follow youngsters like this for a long time while they are allowed to have small amounts of the food that has caused a frightening reaction in the past but has been shown to be tolerated recently during challenges until we are persuaded that it is really safe for them to eat the food in question. It should be pointed out that a positive skin test, in a circumstance like this, may persist long beyond the time that the food can be shown to cause problems and, therefore, the skin test itself is not a diagnostic test that will assure proper identification of foods causing problems when they are eaten.

Tammy was fourteen months old when we began following her. She had a history of chronic diarrhea defined as abnormal stools continuously for more than six weeks. She had undergone many dietary manipulations without identifying a cause for her problem. Perhaps because of the chronic diarrhea, and also because of the many food manipulations, Tammy was small for her age. Her parents were concerned about her poor weight gain, and this was one of the reasons they came to see us. We began by placing her on a very strict elimination diet using an elemental formula. Her diarrhea quickly resolved, and over the next two months we were able to demonstrate that when she consumed dairy products or soy protein, her profuse diarrhea returned. She did not have a convincing positive skin test to those foods. We followed Tammy for several years, and by her third birthday she no longer reacted to either milk or soy, being able to consume both these foods in usual quantities.

Comments: Tammy illustrates a group of children who have what are called protein enteropathies. The food is able to damage the intestine in a way that researchers have not been able to define at this time. The most common foods producing this reaction are wheat, which produces a condition called celiac disease, milk, and soy. A few other foods including foods commonly on the elimination diet (p. 39), such as chicken and rice, have also been associated with these reactions. Except for the enteropathy associated with wheat, or more specifically the gluten fraction of wheat, these children seem to improve by about the time of their third birthday. The mechanism in these children does not seem to involve the antibodies detected by skin tests, and, in fact, their skin tests are usually negative.

Beth was seven years old when we first met her, and she had a seven-year history of florid eczema. Nothing ever seemed to control her eczema very well, but it clearly had periods of waxing and waning. Although she had had an allergy evaluation in the past, the results were equivocal with regard to her diet. Beth was placed on a strict elimination diet such as that illustrated in this book, and her skin was treated intensively with creams and hydration. After the skin had improved, skin testing was undertaken and she was found to have positive skin tests to wheat, milk, eggs, walnuts, soy, and shrimp. Since most of these foods, except for the nuts and eggs, were not under suspicion, they were reintroduced openly into the diet. Double-blind food challenges demonstrated that her eczema was clearly aggravated by peanuts, walnuts, and eggs.

Comments: There has long been a controversy about the potential for eczema to be triggered by foods. Recent research has demonstrated rather unequivocally that in some, but not all, children with eczema, foods play an important role and food elimination diets followed by the proper challenges are important in making the diagnosis.

Lawrence was a forty-five-year-old gentleman who came to us after having been seen in a local emergency room with a severe reaction characterized by abdominal cramping, vomiting, diarrhea, lowering of blood pressure, a feeling of chest tightness, and hoarseness. This occurred immediately following a meal at which the primary constituent was shrimp. He reported having eaten shrimp many times in the past and was puzzled by this association. He denied having exercised immediately before or after that meal. Skin testing with shrimp and associated shellfish was completely negative. During extensive discussion, it was decided that we would carefully and over a period of time challenge him to shrimp. Much to our amazement, he was eventually able to consume ten shrimp at a single serving without any reaction.

Comments: This case illustrates observations for which we do not have an explanation and that cause many allergists to lie awake at night wondering what type of advice to give patients like Lawrence. We have seen a number of patients like this, and when we were unable to reproduce their reaction to shellfish, I've told them that very carefully and with epinephrine handy and someone who can take them to the nearest emergency room, they could carefully try to eat shrimp. The problem is that while there is a strong association between the shrimp ingestion and the severe reaction, proof of cause and effect is lacking. Our inability to reproduce the symptoms during either open or blind challenges, suggests that something else is causing the reaction. Patients, such as Lawrence, could have suffered from food intoxication, i.e., food poisoning, but it usually does not cause chest and throat symptoms, but rather gastrointestimal symptoms. The point about exercise is important, since it has recently been shown that severe reactions such as the one described can occur after the ingestion of certain foods, followed by vigorous exercise. This is a list that has been expanding in the last few years. Usually these people have a history that they have eaten a particular food and then exercised vigorously. Most of the time there is a positive skin test for the food causing the problems. There have been a few patients reported in whom eating apparently any meal followed within two hours by exercise will cause a frightening reaction.

Mark was twenty-eight years old and had a history of asthma in childhood but had not been troubled for many years. Following a respiratory infection about one year prior to our meeting him, his asthma had recurred and had been a mild, but annoying, problem, especially following exercise in the cold. He reported that twice in the preceding three months he had eaten at friends' houses and afterwards had had episodes of marked vomiting and asthma. Our initial investigation was aimed toward identifying things in these environments he might have inhaled that would produce asthma episodes, but the vomiting did seem to be a puzzling symptom. Evaluation of the meals suggested that on both of these occasions he had ingested soy protein. Double-blind challenges were undertaken, and we were able to reproduce both the vomiting and asthma symptoms, including objective measurements of his asthma symptoms by a device called a pulmonary function machine. His skin test to soy protein was positive.

Comments: This case illustrates a less common presentation of food allergy producing gastrointestinal and respiratory symptoms. Mark had apparently been able to eat soy without a problem for many years, and what caused his change in both his asthma and gastrointestinal symptoms is not clear to us at the present time. One interesting food that has been reported but not seen by us to cause similar kinds of symptoms is celery. Exactly what the mechanism is by which celery can produce these symptoms is a puzzle.

Children in the first two years of life are often subjected to dietary alterations. Most symptoms that young children experience have elicited inquiries about possible associations with food. One or more foods are often removed from the diet, and the symptoms resolve. The dietary exclusion may persist for months or even years before the food is returned to the diet. It is unnecessary for the majority of these children to be seen by an allergist, but an approach that shortens the dietary exclusion is recommended. Most of the symptoms are transient and usually not related to foods. If the presumed reaction is not severe, then after the symptoms have resolved, the food should be reintroduced into the diet, starting with small amounts. If the reaction is reproduced, then the challenges should be repeated every one to three months, depending on the severity of the reaction. Experience has shown that even the foods that do cause reactions can usually be placed back in the diet within a few months of the original diagnosis, thus greatly shortening the time of exclusion for foods that are offenders. This makes life much easier for busy mothers and fathers who have things to do besides preparing special meals. It also makes a developing tot who cannot understand dietary limitations less difficult to feed.

Children whose food reactions are severe or who continue to react for prolonged periods will benefit from evaluation by an allergist, who can determine the degree of sensitivity, arrange careful food challenges, and discuss the prognosis.

DISCLAIMER

The examples presented in chapter 5 represent composite histories obtained numerous times from many different patients. The food challenges and results thereof accurately reflect the procedure exactly as performed. Any resemblance of these examples to specific individuals is purely coincidental.

VI

How to Do It at Home

Over the years many people have asked me if I would write down how food allergy or, more properly, suspicions of adverse reactions to foods could be evaluated by individuals at home. In general, I do *not* recommend the do-it-yourself approach to medical problems, because I think certain situations can be dangerous. However, there are circumstances in which it is possible for people with mild or vague symptoms that might be associated with food ingestion to test themselves *carefully* at home. The following comments are *absolutely not designed* for the evaluation of any problem that might, in any remote way, be *life-threatening or trigger severe symptoms,* either those that have been previously associated with food ingestion or are strongly suspected of being associated with food ingestion.

The most important principle to remember is that you must want to determine whether the food is really a problem. A little thought given to the problem of the association between the symptoms and food ingestion will strongly suggest to most people that the first thing to do is make the symptoms go away, and the easiest way to do that is to eliminate suspected foods. What if, as many patients say, they suspect something in the diet is a problem but they don't have any idea of what it might be? In those circumstances, the easiest thing to do is to use an elimination diet, and one is provided in the primer on page 39. It will quickly be seen that this diet is really a modification of most of the standard chicken, rice, and vegetable diets that have long been used and have gone under many names. This particular diet is a modification of the one that we have used for many years. (The

ELIMINATION DIET

Food Permitted

Rice in any form
(Rice cakes and rice cereal especially helpful)

Pineapple
Apricots
Cranberries
Peaches
Pears
Apples
} also canned fruit and juices of these

Lamb
Chicken
Asparagus
Beets
Carrots
Lettuce
Sweet Potatoes

White Vinegar
Olive Oil
Honey
Cane or Beet Sugar
Salt
Safflower Oil

Avoid all foods not on this list.

This is *not* a nutritionally complete diet and must only be used without the advice of a physician or nutritionist for short periods (two weeks or less).

diet is not nutritionally complete and thus should not be used for more than two weeks!)

In general, the diet should be undertaken for about one week. At the end of this time, you should have a fairly clear idea of whether or not foods in the diet are causing symptoms, because if foods are a problem, the symptoms should have disappeared. Since the diet is a nuisance and rather obnoxious, particularly when used with children, any improvement should be viewed as a possible association between the elimination of one or more foods and the disappearance of the symptoms. The more the symptoms persist when the elimination diet is used, the less likely it is that the symptoms are related to something eaten. If at the end of a week there is not a clear answer and you think that perhaps the diet has helped, then it is useful to continue it for another five to seven days. If at the end of fourteen days the diet has not clearly produced a dramatic benefit, it is highly unlikely that diet is the problem. As can be seen from perusal of the diet, the more closely foods are to their natural state, the less one has to be concerned with preservatives, additives, et cetera. The ultimate elimination diet, called an elemental diet, can be used in those circumstances in which it is suspected, rarely, that foods on this elimination diet are causing problems. We have seen problems with both chicken and rice in the rare patient, but in those children it was not a mystery that those foods were a problem. Elemental diets should be used under the supervision of a physician.

Improvement in symptoms following the administration of elimination diet is only step one in determining whether or not diet is the problem. If one stops with improvement and leaves multiple foods out of the diet, one would be doing a disservice both to him/herself or the child and is likely to have acquired the incorrect answer. Again, it must be stressed that elimination of multiple foods may have adverse nutritional consequences and must be avoided.

The next step in most circumstances is the reintroduction of the suspected food into the diet or, if an elimination diet has been used, the reinstitution of a normal diet. This is because in the vast majority of circumstances, especially with young children but also with persons of all ages, the problem for which the diet was being used has disappeared and the symptoms no longer are a problem. Clearly, if this is the case, a prolonged elimination diet is both a nuisance and potentially hazardous from a nutritional point of view. Obviously, if the symptoms do not recur, the problem is solved and one can get on with normal activities and be happy not to have to think about dietary matters any further.

Suppose the symptoms do recur when the foods are reintroduced into the diet. In general, it would be my strongest recommendation that the patient consult with someone who is both qualified and interested in undertaking accurate food challenges. At this point it should be noted that there are many persons who claim an interest in dealing with food problems and who may even claim to be nutritionists. In general, you would be best advised to begin with a *board-certified allergist,* who is prepared to undertake double-blind challenges.

If you are inclined to continue attempting to unravel the problem without professional help, then the next step would be to go back on the elimination diet and allow the symptoms to disappear again. This may mean eliminating one, two, or more foods or using the elimination diet as discussed above. When the symptoms have resolved, then you begin adding foods back into the diet by food group. For example, you can begin with dairy products, if they are not suspected, or one grain at a time or beef or nuts. These large categories are re-added to the diet at two-to-four-day intervals, depending on suspicions that you may have about the food culprits and timing until symptoms begin. At this point it becomes very important to maintain some accurate records. This would include noting the time of onset and character of any symptoms that occur in association with the newly added food. If a food seems to cause symptoms, it should then be removed from the diet and, when the symptoms have again re-

HOME ADVERSE FOOD REACTION EVALUATION

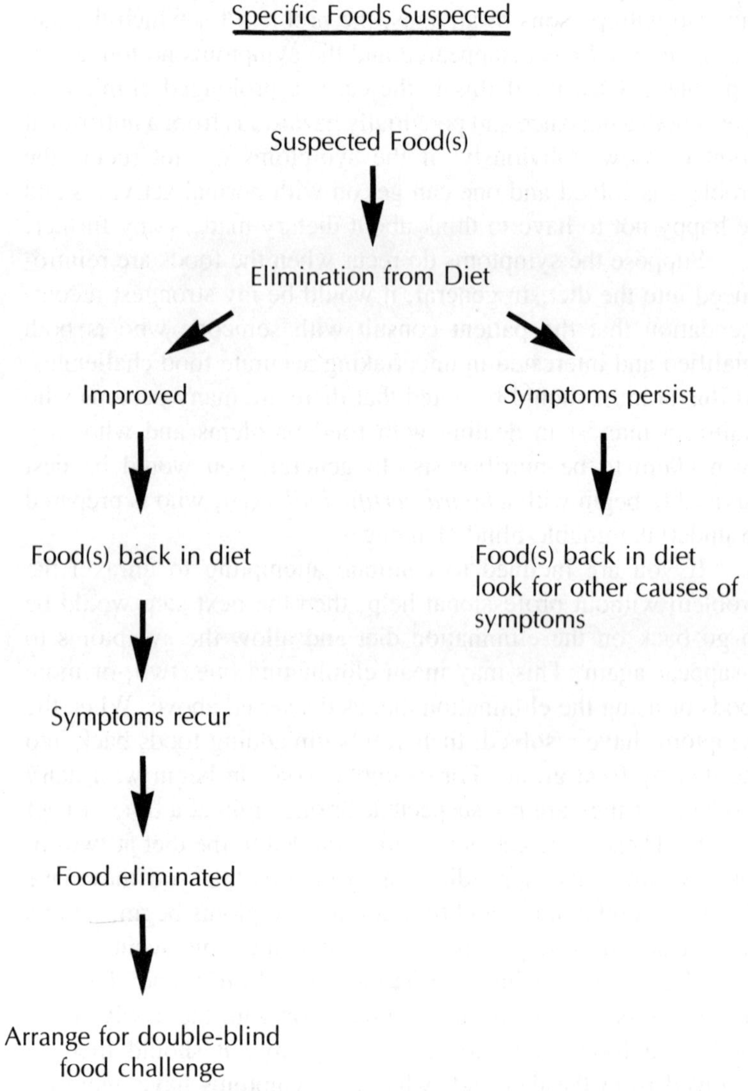

HOME ADVERSE FOOD REACTION EVALUATION

Diet Suspected of Being a Problem—No Specific Food

Elimination Diet (p. 39)

→ Symptoms disappear
Back to regular diet

- → Symptoms recur
  → Back on elimination diet
  → Symptoms disappear
  → Add 1 food at a time at 2–4 day intervals
    - → Symptoms do not appear
      → Leave food in diet—and add another
      → List of tolerated foods
    - → Symptoms appear
      → Remove that food recording timing, symptoms, et cetera on a list, when better—add another food
      → List of problem foods
- → Symptoms do not recur, problem disappeared

→ Symptoms persist
→ Back to regular diet investigate other causes for symptom

solved, another food is added. Any food that does not cause symptoms in two-to-four days is highly unlikely to cause symptoms and should be left in the diet. After this type of testing, you should have two lists: one long list of foods that are tolerated and one short list of one, two, or perhaps three foods which are not tolerated. Any time the list of foods not tolerated becomes excessively long, you should be very suspicious that the observations are incorrect. Controlled scientific studies in both adults and children of all ages strongly suggest that multiple food reactions are the distinct exception rather than the rule. This contradicts most information in other lay publications, but a quiet perusal of the world's double-blind food challenges gives the information that I have just described.

At this stage, when you have the two lists, it is still my firm opinion that double-blind food challenges are appropriate. This is because in almost all studies that have been undertaken, far fewer than 50 percent of suspected histories can be confirmed by double-blind challenges. Why is this important one might ask? The answer is simple. Life seems to be complicated enough without having to worry about the ingestion of foods that are not symptom producers. This is especially true for children who are subjected to long lists of foods that they need to avoid. Despite parents' best efforts, children's peer interactions often place them in an awkward position. It may be a comfort to the parents that Johnny can recite a list of foods that cause him to misbehave, but Johnny will be teased, often unmercifully, by his peers when they are eating favorite foods that he is denied. This often places Johnny in a situation of giving in to peer pressure, especially if he does not believe that the food causes the problem, but then has him in the position of being dishonest with this parents. In my opinion, this is to be avoided. The circumstance with adults is a bit different in that most adults who avoid multiple foods usually cope fairly well and don't mind the annnoyance. A large number of the patients that we see have been subjected to elimination diets that they find impossible to follow and, therefore, have appealed to us to find out the correct answer.

A couple of examples may clarify the use of the diet. Colicky babies are notorious for major disruptions in households. Unfortunately, most of these compact Jekyll and Hydes do not have food allergy, but some do. It is easy and occasionally vastly rewarding to find those who do. The procedure is simple and relatively inexpensive. Take the little darling off all foods and substitute one of the elemental formulas, such as Nutramigen®which may be found in the pharmacy section of most large grocery stores. (Pediatricians and family physicians are familiar with this diet.) Since the formula is nutritionally complete, it can be used as the sole diet for prolonged periods. If the colic is due to a food in the diet, deafening quiet should descend upon the household in twenty-four to forty-eight hours. If this occurs, wait a few days and reintroduce the previous formula and foods into the diet one at a time at two-or-three day intervals to see if screaming reappears. Recurrence of the noise suggests the diet is a problem, and I strongly suggest consultation with the child's doctor at this point. Interestingly, it has been found that quite a few of these colicky babies with food-induced symptoms have a positive skin test to the food causing the problem. Unfortunately, this information is not known to many primary physicians, who will tell you that allergy testing in young children is useless. (See chapter 3.)

A second example might be the investigation of symptoms less specific than mentioned above. Headaches are hard to evaluate because they are hard to measure, but many people do associate some of their headaches with food consumption. This example concerns the person with frequent headaches but no food association, as opposed to the person with occasional headaches strongly associated with specific foods. To examine the possible association between the diet and frequent headaches, use the strict elimination diet. While the diet is being followed, maintain a daily diary of the headaches (timing, duration, character) and also record food infractions (cheating on the diet). If the headache pattern doesn't change, the diet is unlikely to be the culprit. If it does change, then begin reintroducing foods into the diet at three-to-four day intervals to see if the headache pattern worsens. The headache diary should be continued. Begin by introducing foods that will quickly make the diet more palatable: wheat, beef, corn, et cetera. If a food is in the diet for three-to-four days without causing problems, leave it in; if the symptom frequency increases, remove the last food added and note it as a possible culprit. When the process is complete you should have two lists: a short one with incriminated foods and a long one with tolerated foods. At this point, double-blind challenges are strongly advised to eliminate biases that will have developed during the elimination-reintroduction process. An allergist experienced in the use of food challenges will be essential.

There are some blind food challenges that can actually be undertaken at home, and the more resourceful the family, the more of these that can be performed. Again, it is to be stressed that if the child is suspected of having severe or life-threatening symptoms, food challenge is a potentially dangerous, hazardous practice and absolutely is not to be undertaken except under medical supervision. The most entertaining problems to challenge at home have been the behavior problems. We and some of our families have had a very entertaining time hiding foods from a child and one parent so that objective observations can be made. Let me provide a common example, which is very easy to undertake. Suppose, as seems to be the current rage in our society, sugar is suspected of making Johnny's behavior obnoxious. We want to test this hypothesis at a time when any change in Johnny's behavior will be particularly noticed. Therefore, a very useful time to do this is on a Saturday or Sunday afternoon, when Johnny's father is hoping to have peace while watching an important ball game. Since there seem to be important ball games at all times of the year, there is almost no time of the year when this cannot be undertaken. Mother reports to the father that he will be the baby-sitter for the afternoon and that she is headed off to do the family shopping. Just before she goes, she places lunch on the table. The best place to hide a fair quantity of sugar is in hamburgers. I have often suggested to mothers that they take the amount of sugar that they think is likely to produce problems and put it in the youngster's hamburger. It is highly unlikely that most youngsters will pay any attention to the altered taste, especially given the amount of catsup they put on their hamburgers. Once the hamburger has been served, Johnny's mother immediately disappears, making every effort to not reveal the fact that something unusual is taking place. When she returns from her shopping trip, one of two things will be happening. Father will be watching the end of the ball game, and peace will be reigning over the home. If this is not the situation, father will be scraping Johnny from the ceiling or off the wall and will be in a foul humor because the ball game has been so frequently interrupted by Johnny's misbehavior. Although this is not a very scientific way to acquire an answer, it certainly, if properly undertaken, is the truest form of blind food challenge, and Johnny, who has been eating the food, and his father, who made the observations, have no idea that something has happened. In our small series of families, we have yet to find that sugar or other suspected foods that have been given in the above manner have produced symptoms, and this has eliminated from consideration many of the annoying dietary prohibitions that families have been using.

This is not to say that in certain situations Johnny's behavior is not unpleasant; it just reveals that the diet is not the source of the unpleasantness. Patients have often said to me, "Well, if the food is not the problem, what is the problem?" I have declined to speculate in many circumstances, but there is one set of circumstances that seems most frequently associated with problems. Observations about children's unruly behavior often occurs at times of holidays, such as Christmas or Easter, when grandparents are on the scene and large amounts of candy are being consumed. It is highly unlikely and probably sacrilegious for anyone to blame

Christmas for a child's misbehavior. Blaming grandparents causes a major family upheaval and often eliminates the major source of expensive-name-brand children's clothes, which grandparents seem much more likely than parents to purchase. Therefore, the obvious offender must be the evil sugar/chocolate manufacturers, and, therefore, these foods are eliminated. The stronger the prohibition is made, the more likely it seems that a self-fulfilling prophecy will occur, and since each time Johnny consumes candy he is expected to behave like a brat, that is the observed outcome.

I do not want to leave the impression that I think that it wouldn't be nice if children's behavior could be modified easily by changing the diet. As I have observed earlier in this chapter, the occasional infant with colic will have his/her behavior dramatically changed by dietary elimination. Unfortunately, behavioral matters are generally more complicated than a simple dietary solution will provide. Again, in those instances in which children's behavior seems dramatically modifed by diet, I urge parents to consider the psychological implications of elimination diets for their children and to have their observations confirmed by double-blind food challenges.

An important caution: Never, never, never should any children or adults test themselves with any food that may have caused a serious reaction. If there is <u>any</u> doubt about the potential danger of any food, a physician <u>must</u> be consulted. Death can result from the ingestion of a food to which a person is highly allergic!

VII

Treatment and Prognosis

TREATMENT

At the present time, the only truly effective treatment for a confirmed food sensitivity is elimination of the food from the diet. I have been asked how to explain an elimination diet to a three-year-old who sees people eating things he cannot eat. This is not an easy task, and I have suggested approaching it in two ways. First, the situation should be explained to the child as simply as possible, relating in concrete terms what has happened in the past when the food was eaten. The second approach has been for the family to adhere to the special diet as much as possible in the child's presence. Treats that have been prohibited should not be eaten by parents and older siblings in front of the child. Finally, parents often have insights into handling this problem that the doctor does not possess and are often very successful at helping children cope with this problem. Some cities have good support groups, especially those with a chapter of the Asthma and Allergy Foundation of America.

Although many therapies have been tried, most of these have not been shown to be effective in instances where the food sensitivity has been objectively confirmed. A number of drugs have been administered to patients having adverse reactions to foods, including antihistamines, cromolyn, a drug that prevents the release of the chemical mediators, and cortisone-containing drugs. In the vast majority of cases, these medications have not yet been shown to be helpful.

Most patients having a food sensitivity have one or perhaps two foods that they cannot eat without harm. This makes it relatively easy to contrive a nutritionally and aesthetically palatable diet for these patients. Our experience has been that it is unusual, except in small children, for there to be multiple food sensitivities. When this does occur in small children, it is not difficult to provide a diet that is nutritionally acceptable.

A number of attempts has been made to "desensitize" patients who have food sensitivity. This has been performed by the administration of injections, drops under the tongue, and small amounts of extract, which are swallowed. Immunological principles make this a highly appealing idea; however, at the present time, it has not been objectively demonstrated to be useful. (See chapter 8.)

PROGNOSIS

It has often been said that children outgrow their food sensitivity. Yet this question has only recently been examined carefully enough to determine whether or not this occurs. Certainly, one sees adults who have been noted to have food sensitivity for many years. In a study of children using double-blind food challenges, it was found that children less than three years of age at the time the diagnosis is made are much more likely to "outgrow" the adverse reaction that was originally noted than are those who are beyond their third birthday. In fact, the majority of foods originally proven to produce symptoms by double-blind food challenge continue to produce symptoms for many years or else are carefully avoided. In all age groups, the foods most likely to stop producing reactions are milk, eggs, and soy. Specifically, 44 percent of positive food challenges in children less than three years of age were negative at the time a subsequent evaluation was conducted one to five years after the original investigation. In children beyond their third birthday, 19 percent of the originally positive food challenges are now negative. One would conclude that while some children do "outgrow" their symptomatic sensitivity to food, many do not, and in those the problem is likely to persist for years.

The most important approach to patients with either suspected or proven adverse reactions to foods is frequent rechallenge with the suspected foods. By the time you have reached this part of this book, you should he persuaded that many reactions attributed to foods are the result of coincidence or may have been transient. Therefore, careful reintroduction of a small amount of the food at regular intervals will determine if the problem continues or is transient. The object of rechallenge is not to make you ill, but to determine if avoidance of the suspected food continues to be necessary. Any food reaction that has been previously confirmed by blind food challenge should only be challenged under medical supervision. The challenge intervals can be every one to three months or up to one year, depending on the food, severity of reaction, and number of times the symptoms have been reproduced. Whenever possible, the rechallenges need to be double-blind (unless an open challenge is negative). Blind rechallenges are important because the more often a reaction has been reproduced, the more strongly held is the belief that the food will cause problems.

Prospects for a "cure" for true food sensitivity at the moment remain as remote as a "cure" for cat allergy and ragweed allergic rhinitis (hay fever). Research now and in the future is aimed toward control and manipulation of the immune system so that the immune system itself can be used to decrease or prevent the adverse reactions. Great care must be used in manipulating the human immune system, because it consists of a complex network of interacting parts. Artificial disruption of one part could disrupt the entire network.

Feeding the Infant of Allergic Parents

An important question is often asked by pregnant mothers

concerning what they themselves should eat and how they should feed their newborns. This is a most intriguing subject, which is the focus of important current research. Unfortunately, at the present time we do not have an exact answer. Rather than review all of the research that has tried to define a proper maternal and newborn diet, I will instead offer a set of recommendations that are based upon this reasearch and serve as a reasonable approach for the present and the next few years while better answers are sought. Not every pediatrician and family physician will agree with these suggestions, and they are meant to serve as guidelines rather than dogmatic instructions.

The following recommendations are meant for families with a history of allergy and *not* for the general population. This means that someone in the family who is a close relative of the baby has signficant allergy, including one or more of the following: asthma, allergic rhinitis (hay fever), eczema, and food allergy. The history seems to be most significant when the symptoms occur in one or both parents or in a sibling. It has been found that if one parent has allergy, the newborn has a 30 to 50 percent chance of developing allergic problems in the first few years. If both parents have an allergic history, the baby has a 60 to 90 percent chance of developing allergic problems. (These numerical ranges are quite broad because many different studies have been performed and have shown rather different results.)

I recommend the following:

1. The pregnant mother should maintain a normal diet, because several good studies have not shown that limiting the maternal diet has a significant impact on the development of allergy in the baby. Limiting the mother's diet could result in nutritional compromise for both mother and baby.
2. The infant should be breast-fed for at least six months if at all possible. When a supplement is required, one of the elemental formulas (such as Nutramigen) should be used.

3. The nursing mother should avoid consuming eggs, dairy products, and peanuts. (This does not include peanut oil.)
4. The introduction of solid foods into the infant's diet should be delayed according to the following schedule:
   a. 6–12 months: vegetables, rice, meat, noncitrus fruits
   b. 12–18 months: dairy, wheat, citrus, corn, soy
   c. 24 months: egg
   d. 36 months: peanut and fish

With luck, these measures may prevent the onset of allergic symptoms, but most studies show that feeding programs such as the one outlined here are more likely to delay the onset of allergic symptoms rather than prevent them altogether.

VIII

Controversial Procedures and Techniques

The following discussion presents the author's information and opinions about some of the commonly performed procedures that have not been shown to be valid when examined using the scientific method as described earlier in this primer.

FOOD TESTING

Sublingual food drops

Sublingual food drops have been used in testing patients thought to have adverse reactions to foods. In this test, patients sit in a chair and drops of various kinds of food solutions are placed under the tongue. A symptom score is then kept by an observer who scores any type of behavioral, respiratory, or skin symptom that the patient manifests. This procedure has generally been undertaken in an uncontrolled fashion with neither the patient nor the observer blinded to the substance being used. Observations have been largely subjective. No published properly controlled study exists that associates the results of sublingual food testing with double-blind food challenges in order to show some correlation between the observations made during the sublingual challenge and the patient's ingestion to the food.

Titration Neutralization Food Skin Testing

This is another controversial procedure, which has generally not been performed blindly and is based on the unproven idea that injection of material into the skin in varying concentrations will allow one to find a dose that, when given regularly to the patient, will neutralize symptoms related to food ingestion. This has also been known as the Rinkel technique. A very elaborate procedure, it is the subject of lengthy books and articles. The same critical comment may be applied to this as to sublingual food drops. Studies have attempted to correlate the associations drawn between observations made using this technique and various kinds of ingestion tests. It is the author's opinion that these have not been properly controlled by being performed in a double-blind manner and the results have been subject to the bias of the person performing the investigation. At the present time, this constitutes a very expensive and somewhat uncomfortable procedure for which there is still no proven efficacy.

Cytotoxic Food Testing

Recently, this particular technique has gained a great following and has been widely proposed around the country and used by many people who are not trained as allergists. Blood is drawn from a patient, the white cells are placed in little wells in a tray, and then various food extracts are added to these wells. The patient's white cells are observed through a microscope and scored according to how they react. These tests are very expensive, and the studies that have attempted to correlate the observations of the white cells with true adverse reactions to foods in patients have not been successful at showing this association. Despite this, it is still a widely used technique. One of the cautions that the author would propose to any patient considering this testing is that it is rare, if not unheard of, for a patient who has undergone this technique to be told that he or she is entirely normal. According to the proponents of this technique, almost everyone has some food allergy. The patients who undergo this procedure are frequently given a long list of foods that they should avoid or eat in a special rotation, along with some very expensive vitamins. The patients are told that they will certainly feel better. Obviously, there is a great deal of suggestion associated with a fancy and expensive test and the assurance from a physician or other healer that the patient's health will improve. This may be considered an example of healing that lacks scientific support.

Since the publication of the first edition of this book, a number of individuals have made buckets of money charging people large sums of money for treatment based on this unproven procedure. At this time, the federal government, through its Medicare and Medicaid programs, has finally stopped spending your tax dollars on this procedure, and many insurance companies will no longer pay for these tests. One state has even prosecuted some proponents of the test for practicing medicine without a license. However, many of the practitioners using this procedure are resourceful entrepreneurs and have found a new approach, which they call the "food immune complex test." This test sounds even more impressive because its idea is based on sound scientific findings. *BUT*, it is a test that is being applied to daily problems, and it ignores the fact that most of us have "food immune complexes" in our blood. A food immune complex is a combination between the protein of a food we eat and an antibody against the food. At present, we do not know how to use the results of this test to diagnose and treat individuals who may have adverse reactions to foods. The test and results from it should be regarded as experimental at this time.

CONTROVERSIAL TREATMENT FOR FOOD ALLERGY

Food Injections

In some areas of the country, patients are receiving injections for food just as they might receive injections for ragweed allergic rhinitis (hay fever) or other inhalant allergy. Once again, while the idea of being able to give someone injections and reduce their sensitivity to foods seems appealing, no properly controlled studies exist that show this procedure to be effective. Again, a great deal of room for the power of positive thinking and positive suggestion lies in these areas. These injections tend to be expensive, and often the patient is told that treatment will need to continue for years. It should be emphasized, as discussed earlier, that those few foods to which a patient truly has an adverse reaction should be avoided, with the undertaking of periodic challenges, until it becomes clear that the patient's sensitivity is going to be long-term or it has resolved.

Dietary Therapy

A number of diets are currently in vogue to treat various kinds of problems. The primary ones, receiving the greatest amount of attention, are diets that eliminate food additives and preservatives (the Feingold diet) and diets that eliminate all "refined" sugar. These diets have some very enthusiastic proponents, and parents' groups actually meet and help each other in the application of these diets. Careful studies, particularly of the Feingold diet, have rarely been able to reproduce the findings in any children that Feingold and others have described in nearly all their cases. The conclusion at the present time would be that while a few children scattered about the country may *truly* benefit from this diet, the problem is small rather than as vast as the proponents claim. Many patients have benefited from the diet; however, it cannot be emphasized too strongly that the benefit is not one of cause and effect based on the diet, but rather is one based on conviction that the diet will help. Once again, it is to be stressed that this constitutes healing and not the application of scientific medicine. Certainly, there is nothing wrong with healing nor with the improvement that families find when these diets are used; however, this has certain implications for the broad public health. If regulatory decisions are based on opinion, testimonials, and anecdotes without properly performed studies, it may cost everyone more money without providing any health benefits. Food allergy is a medical problem in some individuals rather than a public health problem that may affect anyone.

As has been typical in this arena, a new "revolutionary" concept has come on the scene since the first edition of this book was written—"the Yeast-hypersensitivity Syndrome." Instead of sugar, additives, and preservatives being the culprit responsible for all of man's ills, it is the yeast called candida, which we all carry in our intestinal tract. The list of symptoms attributed to this insidious yeast is truly startling, but most of these symptoms are subjective. The treatment is long, arduous, and expensive. Once again, vast claims are made without any scientific proof, but a gullible public is spending millions on treatments for this problem.

Some physicians who treat food allergy use a rotation diet (also called a rotary diversified diet). It is based on the principle that some patients will not have reactions to food that they eat infrequently or with a specified interval between exposures. This diet has often been used for people who are thought to have "delayed" food allergy. It makes some sense if viewed from the perspective of trying to keep the total dose (exposure) of a food below a specific total quantity during a certain time interval. Different physicians use the diet differently. Generally, patients are allowed to eat troublesome foods at only a defined numer of meals during each week. Sometimes the foods are allowed three consecutive days each week.

Unfortunately, the vast majority of patients subjected to this form of therapy have never had their food reaction proven by objective means. Thus it is impossible to determine whether or not reported benefits are due to a change in the frequency of consumption of the food or to the placebo effect.

In my opinion, the application of elimination diets, especially for long periods of time, is not entirely benign. When treating children who have been on these diets and discussing with them their feelings about the requirement for the diet, I have been surprised to learn that the children have very strong feelings about the need for this treatment and how it makes them different from their peers. Parents must consider the effect on their child, who may think, *I am bad, there is something wrong with me, and the only way I can be controlled is with a special diet. I am not able to eat the things that my friends can eat, because I am sick.* Parents often get very agitated about children's need for continuous medication, and yet the effect of dietary changes does not evoke the same kind of concern.

We need to ask ourselves if we are creating new eating disorders with all our diet fads. Certainly, children with true food sensitivity do display aversions to those foods and even when they outgrow the problem they are unwilling to eat the food. Our society is already very food-conscious, and we are seeing increasing numbers of young people with definable eating disorders (anorexia, bulimia). Is our obsession with food allergy going to create new and equally troublesome problems, or are we going to become more critical in our acceptance of the claims of every purveyor of a new diet or idea about food and health?

Wouldn't it be nice if the proponents of the procedures discussed in chapter 8 admitted that they are experimental techniques and undertook studies to demonstrate this efficacy? Everyone would benefit.

Afterword

One of Webster's definitions of primer is "a textbook which presents the first principles of a subject." This primer has been written to acquaint the reader with the principles and practice of the evaluation of food allergy. It is hoped that the primer will serve as a bridge between the confusion in much of the lay "health" literature and the complexities of the medical literature. The interested reader will be able to pursue the details of the subject by consulting the additional readings. The primer is purposely short so that the reader can grasp the important points without becoming mired in the repetitious claims and explanations characteristic of many of the "health tomes."

A few important points need to be stressed as messages to the reader. First are the principles of the scientific method, which distinguish unbiased evaluation from healing based on belief. Second are the principles encompassed by the difference between symptomatic and asymptomatic food sensitivity, including interpretation of skin testing. Third is the use of double-blind food challenges, and fourth is the proper treatment and ongoing evaluation.

The medical profession has lost some of its mystique in the last two decades, and patients have begun to question physicians about diagnosis and treatment. With chronic illness as a continuing frontier in medicine, the critical questioning is laudable but often becomes unpleasant. This can be avoided by having the doctor and patient work together to unravel a problem without it becoming an adversarial proceeding. The physician must be willing to explain pros and cons of the evaluation process and treatment so that they are clear to the patient. The patient needs to be responsible for understanding his illness and carrying out measures required for his or her own health maintenance.

A continuing and critical evaluation of the problems that plague us will bring light to areas of darkness without passionate belief interfering with progress. This is especially important when dealing with adverse reactions to foods.

Glossary

ALLERGY. An adverse reaction to a substance that may occur following exposure to inhaled, ingested or injected substances and involves one or more components of the immune system.

ANAPHYLAXIS. Specific sensitivity to a substance acquired on a previous exposure so that a subsequent exposure results in a severe reaction.

ANTIBODIES. Protein molecules formed by the body as a very specific response to antigens.

ANTIGENS. Molecules, usually proteins, that have the property of stimulating the immune system to produce a response.

ASYMPTOMATIC SENSITIVITY. A condition in which there are detectable antibodies to a food but no symptoms during exposure. (see p. 4.)

COLIC. A condition that occurs in infants and is characterized by crying, fretfulness, poor sleeping, drawing up the legs, and other signs of irritability and discomfort.

DOUBLE-BLIND FOOD CHALLENGE. Test utilizing administration of a suspected food so that neither the patient nor the observer is aware of the food being ingested.

ECZEMA. A scaly skin rash composed of small red and white bumps that are very itchy, leading to scratching, which may be severe enough to produce bleeding and allow skin infections to occur. Also called atopic dermatitis.

ENZYME. A protein that can aid in a biochemical reaction such as the digestion of complex molecules.

IMMUNE COMPLEX. Combination of food protein that has been absorbed into the body and an antibody. (Also called antigen-antibody complex.)

IMMUNE SYSTEM. The collection of organs, cells, and molecules that are responsible for both protective and adverse responses to substances encountered in the environment.

IMMUNOGLOBULINS. Molecules of antibody (see page 3 for details).

IMMUNOGLOBULIN E (IgE). The antibody with the property of attaching to cells and which is responsible for prompt onset reactions.

MAST CELLS. The cells to which IgE attaches and which contain chemicals called mediators, which bring about the reactions resulting in symptoms.

MEDIATORS. Chemicals in various cells that bring about reactions resulting in symptoms.

MUCOSA. The inner layer of cells of the gastrointestinal tract that are closest to the contents in the lumen.

PLACEBO. A substance used in testing that does not have any known physiological effect that might mimic a reaction to the real substance being tested.

SCIENTIFIC METHOD. Evaluation of a problem designed to obtain results uninfluenced by the bias of the investigator or subjects and controlling as many variables as possible.

SYMPTOMATIC SENSITIVITY. Detectable antibodies to a food (or inhaled or injected substance) and symptoms on exposure (see p. 4.)

URTICARIA (HIVES). Raised bumps (usually white surrounded by redness), often referred to as welts, that are very itchy.

Additional Reading

Many readers may want to pursue this subject further by consulting this reference list. These have been selected because of their general or review nature and should be understandable to anyone willing to make the effort. These articles can be found in any medical school library and in most large hospital libraries.

Atkins, F. M., S. S. Steinberg, and D. D. Metcalfe. 1985. Evaluation of immediate adverse reactions to foods in adult patients. I. Correlation of demographic, laboratory, and prick skin test data with response to controlled oral food challenge. II. A detailed analysis of reaction patterns during oral food challenge. *J. Allergy Clin. Immunol* 75: 348, 356.

Bock, S. A. 1982. The natural history of food sensitivity. *J. Allergy Clin. Immunol.* 69: 173.

——— 1985. Natural history of severe reactions to foods in young children. *J. Pediatrics* 107: 676.

——— 1987. Prospective appraisal of complaints of adverse reactions to foods in children during the first three years of life. *Pediatrics* 79: 683.

Bock, S. A., and C. D. May. 1983. Adverse reactions to food due to hypersensitivity. Ch. 64 in *Allergy: Principles and practice*. Edited by E. Middleton, C. Reed, and E. Ellis, St. Louis: C. V. Mosby Co.

Martin, M., and S. A. Bock. 1983. A clinical discussion of food sensitivity. In *Pediatric Update*. Edited by A. J. Moss. New York: Elsevier Biomedical.

Metcalfe, D. D. (ed.). July 1986. *Journal of Allergy and Clinical Immunology* (supplement), *Symposium proceedings on adverse reactions to foods and food additives 78.*

Sampson, H. A. 1983. Role of immediate food hypersensitivity in the pathogenesis of atopic dermatitis. *J. Allergy Clin. Immunol.* 71: 473.

Sampson, H. A., and R. Albergo. 1983. Comparisons of results of skin tests, RAST, and double-blind, placebo-controlled food challenges in children with atopic dermatitis. *J. Allergy Clin. Immunol.* 74: 26.

The following two articles constitute the most thorough, objective evaluation of the Feingold diet to date. It would be worthwhile for the interested reader to review these and form his own opinion.

Harley, J. P., C. G. Matthews, and P. Eichman. 1978. Synthetic food colors and hyperreactivity in children: A double-blind challenge experiment. *Pediatrics* 62: 975.

Harley, J. P., R. S. Ray, L. Tomasi, et. al. 1978. Hyperkinesis and food additives: Testing the Feingold hypothesis. *Pediatrics* 61: 818.